BRYAN WESLEY

First Time Father At Forty

The Pregnancy To Toddler Handbook I Wish I'd Had As A New Dad

First edition

This book was professionally typeset on Reedsy.
Find out more at reedsy.com

I dedicate this book to my father, Jerry. He worked his whole life, stayed strong for as long as he could, and never failed to set the perfect example of what a strong, caring, and loving father should be. You always had an answer to every question. Thanks, Pop.

Contents

Foreword

So, I was forty years old, shaving, looking down at the sink, where my wife had left a surprise for me, that would change my life as I knew it. I'd long ago accepted that we would not have a child because I was forty, and it hadn't happened yet. We had been trying for years, not knowing if it would ever happen for us. Month after month, our hopes were crushed, and ultimately we accepted that perhaps it wasn't in the cards for us. Of course, we would still be happy with each other. In front of me was the first piece of tangible evidence, a positive pregnancy test, giving hope that such a thing was possible.

Thank the Lord for his many blessings, one of which is that I'm not someone who panics, or at least if I am; I channel it into being extremely productive. I wiped off the shaving cream, my bottom lip was quivering involuntarily and with tears filling my eyes I embraced my wife, who sat eagerly on the side of the bed, waiting for my reaction. It was the happiest moment of my life to that point. This journey through parenthood had just started and I knew I had a lot to learn. This book is a collection, a handbook of the things I wish I had when I started my parenting journey.

May your own little miracle be just as happy.

1

Introduction

I'm not a doctor or medical expert. However, I've had training in emergency medicine and provided dispatch medical instructions to help with emergency deliveries until paramedics or more skilled personnel arrived on the scene as an Emergency 911 Dispatcher. Who I am is a father and a son wishing his father was still alive so that I could ask him some fundamental questions. In place of that, I wish I had a book like this to read and find the answers it offers. I am a husband, so I use the term wife. I'm not judging, so substitute the term girlfriend or partner if that fits your situation, but for ease of reading and because this is my book about my experiences, I'll use wife. Expect to find accurate information in this book and the occasional reality check. This book is my experiences, and hard-earned lessons kept intentionally simple and absent excessive medical jargon. I'm too old for hand-holding, but this information will help you get ready for fatherhood. Look for supply lists and checklists, along with some heartfelt shared experiences. I didn't do it all correctly, but I learned from my mistakes. I'm sharing the good and bad with you so you may benefit from my wisdom. Always consult your medical professional on all things health-related. Do whatever you must to protect your family because they are ultimately your responsibility. I wish you Godspeed in doing so.

2

The First 12 weeks

The first 12 weeks, also known as the first trimester, may have already come and gone by the time your wife realizes she's pregnant. Whatever the case, the moment she thinks she's pregnant, it's time to get your mind right. You've got to step up quickly, become a leader, and start making good decisions. Be a responsible adult, and start living for your family. The time for being selfish or thoughtless is over. It's not about you, and it won't be again for a long time. You're about to become a selfless, compassionate, thoughtful, reflective, and active father.

Simply put, if you or your wife smoked, drank, engaged in recreational drug use, or other risky behaviors, you need to knock it off. Draw strength from whatever you need to, tell yourself you're becoming some elevated being, a Father, whatever it takes. Just knock it off. If you can't get by on willpower alone, find help. Support each other, and pull together with your wife, because you'll need each other over the next nine months and the rest of your lives, as you've never needed each other before. Don't be scared; just understand that the situation is serious, and get in the game.

Like never before, you and your wife are Team Baby, and every team needs a leader, so step up and lead. Be the head of the household, and make the decisions required to get your family through to a successful birth and bring your baby home to a prepared house. Of course, teamwork is paramount, but the critical part of that statement is the work, so get ready.

Get informed. Practice OPSEC, or operational security. Simply put, this means that now is not the time for making announcements. You may be nervous or excited, but consider practicing discretion and keeping your mouth shut. Why? The sad truth is that in research from Miles (2021), about 10 percent of known pregnancies end in miscarriage, and more than **80 percent of these losses happen before 12 weeks**. I can tell you from experience that it is already hard enough to ride high for 16 weeks of bliss only to find you've joined the 10 percent club. Then, to make phone calls and share the sad news that you've suffered a terrible loss. If the worst happens, take the time you need to grieve. It's important to get whatever help is necessary to move past it. The longer you can keep the news to yourself or a small circle of confidants, the easier it may be to handle any setbacks. At a minimum, hold it together for 12 weeks, or do yourself a favor and lock it up until you've reached the **18-20 week milestone** and learn the baby's gender. More on that later.

The OBGYN, or Doctor of Obstetrics and Gynecology, is your new best friend. An obstetrician is a doctor who helps the mother leading up to, during, and after childbirth. Your wife's gynecologist may be a practicing obstetrician. If not, you should look for a board-certified obstetrician in your insurance network. That's the criteria I started with when I shopped around on my insurance's website for a doctor. Check the ratings and reviews because that quickly allowed me to disqualify numerous candidates who weren't up to scratch. Find someone you and your wife like, who will answer your questions. If you don't like the first doctor, move on to the next. Also, ask questions, and keep a running list of pending questions in a notes application on your smartphone, so you have them prepared when visiting the doctor. **You'll be visiting the doctor much more frequently as the pregnancy progresses.** Start with questions about conducting certain activities in your daily life. Some activities are risky during pregnancy. Find out what signs of trouble you must look for, and learn to recognize those symptoms by heart. In an emergency, you won't have time to reach for a book or find a list you wrote down on a stray piece of paper if your wife starts spotting or bleeding. Here's one of those lists I mentioned, but again, you need to verify and discuss it with your doctor because things change, and I am not an MD.

- **Vaginal Bleeding or Spotting** is typically the first sign of a miscarriage. However, twenty-five percent of women will find bloody spots on their underwear or toilet tissue early in the pregnancy. Most of these spotting events do not lead to miscarriage. Regardless, contact your healthcare professional or care team without hesitation if bleeding or spotting occurs. You're paying them for this kind of care, and they want to know about it.
- **Abdominal pain:** Shows up as persistent, mild, or sometimes sharp cramps that may present as lower back pain or pressure in the pelvic region; following bleeding. According to Miles (2021b), you should contact your doctor if any pain is experienced anywhere in the abdomen or pelvis during pregnancy. Furthermore, Miles (2021b) states that if the pain is in your wife's shoulders, especially when lying down, call 911 because your wife may be experiencing something called an ectopic pregnancy.

Again, your doctor is your best friend, one paid to answer all questions you have, so make the most of that relationship. Your doctor wants to get you and your family across the finish line, so ask your questions, no matter how stupid you think they are. All that matters is that your baby arrives safely. Vigilance is essential here. So be on alert, and check in with your wife frequently, encouraging her to share what she's experiencing with you. Make sure to ask the doctor about Prenatal Vitamins, the importance of Folic Acid, and DHA, so you're giving your baby their best start in life. Next, determine what your wife should eat and drink and start cooking. That was easy for me as I already did the cooking and a majority of the household chores and cleaning. The doctor will tell you that it's important that your wife drinks lots of water; more on that later, but remember to help her hydrate!

You just became an amateur risk analyst. That's your new hobby. Learn about the risk from your doctor, your new partner in protecting your wife and unborn child, get your tools out, and get busy. Sadly, it's a fact that bad things happen to good people every day, so find out what you can do to minimize risks and get it done. If having alcohol in the house is a temptation for your wife, get rid of it. Do the same with anything else that is not good for your wife or baby. Don't want to deal with giving it away? Throw it out. Just get rid of it. If things around the house need fixing and you're handy, now is the time. If you've got wobbly banisters, windows that don't latch, doors that don't close, take action. If you're not handy, call a contractor for jobs that require one.

The order of the day is clean living. Not just for her, but you. I mentioned getting your mind right and being a leader; that's what this means. Set the example, and quit smoking, drinking, or whatever other foolish thing you used to do that doesn't have any place in a home with or expecting a baby. It wasn't that important, to begin with, I can tell you, and it's easier to give up than you probably think. But, eventually, you will start feeling better, and you won't even miss it. You'll find that you're too busy for these things anyway. If all else fails, get whatever help you need to stop because your wife can't do it or be around it if it exposes her or your baby to second-hand smoke or other harmful situations. Even being around smoke can cause babies to have lower birth weight. Your doctor will be happy to tell you all about these risks. The bottom line is to be supportive. If your wife can't have something, you probably shouldn't either.

Through it, all, have a heart. Your wife is entering an unprecedented period of change in her life. Various hormonal changes may accompany this, and each woman is affected differently. It may come with some fairly significant mood swings. Understand that your wife isn't angry with you, though she may say things to the contrary. The tract I took was primarily to stay quiet and continue doing whatever activity was necessary. I applied repetitive persistence and logic in most every situation. I apologized for any perceived short-coming and took action to improve every situation. My wife was very even-keeled through most of the pregnancy and handled it with tremendous aplomb. So I was pretty fortunate. I pray you are as lucky. If you are adrift in a sea of mood swings, just remember to be patient, calm, and sympathetic to what your wife is experiencing. Her feelings are temporary, and like any storm, they too will pass. Resist all urges to escalate.

3

The Documentarian

Pregnancy Milestones are many and varied. You can talk to your doctor or find an app that can tell you all about how big your baby is at the current point in pregnancy. However, below is an overview of milestones I found most significant.

1-12 weeks - First Trimester

- According to Miles (2021), a study found that the odds of a miscarriage drop to 0.7 percent at ten weeks.

13-26 weeks - Second Trimester

- Somewhere between 18-20 weeks, and possibly a couple of weeks earlier, your doctor may be able to determine the gender of the baby. At this point, discuss with your wife if you are ready to reveal the good news and to whom you will share it.

29-40+ weeks - Third Trimester

- Anything after 37 weeks but before 39 is an early term, but the baby may still do well. However, I understand that doctors prefer babies to stay in utero until 39 weeks.

- Thirty-nine weeks - at this point, the baby is full term and ready for birth.
- Forty-one weeks - Anything after 40 weeks will have the doctor consider inducing labor and is late-term.

Become **"The Documentarian."** What I mean by this is that you should **record everything**. I used a notes app on my smartphone to track everything. Ultimately, I wanted to remember everything. Be realistic about everything to remember, and keep notes on all the details, dates, milestones, doctor visits, and appointments. I was fortunate enough to attend these. Make the time and be involved. Your attendance is critical, especially in the beginning. We received devastating news during the last ultrasound of our first pregnancy. I can't imagine what it would have been like for my wife to deal with that alone. The doctor often asks many questions as to her care, and you may need to help in making some decisions. Be there for each other, whatever it takes. Even if everything goes perfectly, you will want to experience firsthand the joys of your baby's first picture. Work will still be there when the baby comes, and you won't regret missing a little work here and there. Still, you may very well regret not taking the opportunity to get informed about what's going on with your baby or what your wife is going through. Take a lot of pictures along the way. Your wife may not feel particularly photogenic, but don't let that stop you. Always reassure her that she's only growing more beautiful. Everyone needs that confidence boost, and there's nothing wrong with showing affection to someone who may desperately need to feel the embrace of her most trusted and closest friend. Remember to show her you love her because that means much more than simply telling her. Your wife's body is going through a great many changes. They may not all be outwardly visible early on in the pregnancy; however, she is experiencing many hormonal changes and changing feelings. Be sensitive to that, and know that no matter how calm she appears on the surface, underneath, she may be battling a tremendous amount of doubt and insecurity. Again, ask your doctor to know and understand the risks, but sex early in the pregnancy can still be quite pleasant, and you should enjoy that while you can, if safe to do so. Depending on how things go, it could become a reasonably infrequent event later on.

It's never too early to start planning. Understand this, pregnancies and kids are expensive. I hope you've got great insurance and some thousands tucked away in an HSA. It's easy to empty a Health Saving Account when you start making frequent doctor visits and spend time at a birthing facility. Take stock of what you own and the space available to you. Understand you are probably under-estimating the amount of space needed for your baby and related things. Consider that a baby requires a room of their own and likely part of your room. If your experience is similar to ours, your baby needs a portion of the living room for diaper changing and tummy time and about half of your bedroom for a: bottle station, a refrigerator, a microwave, a diaper-changing station, a sidecar bassinet, a dresser of their own for all the onesies and burp-clothes. The lists go on and on. So, knowing that might help you decide to part with some things that you've been holding on to for way too long more easily. Spring-Cleaning is a real thing, and before that stork starts circling the neighborhood, make all the room you can.

Now is the time for **planning and researching**, but I can't stress enough that it is ***not*** the time to buy. At this point, in the first trimester, you don't know the gender of the baby. So you should avoid shopping for gender-specific items. While researching, don't forget to start gift registries at the stores where you would like your friends and family to shop for your baby's gifts. Keep in mind that online stores have gift registries. Do anything you can to make the gift-buying experience of family and friends easier. That will streamline the process for you and your wife to get the things you need. Don't make the mistake of thinking that just because something you need is expensive, nobody will purchase it for you. My wife and I were pleasantly surprised by what our friends and family were willing to buy for us. I'll tell you something else, and it's not the happiest memory. We purchased a stroller/car seat combo online the day after Thanksgiving during our first pregnancy. Things didn't work out, and it sat in our basement until the Lord blessed us with our daughter. It was a nearly six hundred dollar reminder that things don't always go according to our plan. Place large purchase items such as a stroller on a gift registry. When placing items on a registry, add several options from which gift-givers may select that meet your need. Don't make these purchases yourself until a month or so after the baby shower. Gifts have the potential to arrive in the weeks following the baby shower.

When planning for needed items, think end-user-oriented. That is, think of whom will be the primary user of the researched tools. For example, I'm over six feet tall, but my wife is a touch over five feet and three inches. Recommendations were not to purchase a drop-side crib due to the risk of damaging the baby's fingers or other injuries. We lowered our crib mattress as our daughter grew taller and stood up inside the crib to keep her from climbing out. With that, my wife could no longer comfortably reach the sheets when putting our daughter down. I could either flex my handyman skills to build a platform for her to walk up when putting our daughter down at night or spend that time bonding with our daughter. I chose to sing her to sleep, watching her nod off before I put her down for her goodnight. So, keep the end user and what my wife calls 'short people problems' in mind when planning your purchases. Keep your registries marked Private at this point. Remember, you haven't made any announcements about a baby on the way, with this being the first trimester.

A few more words on baby registries because they are handy. Baby registries are a great shopping list and a way to keep track of the things you need to buy when preparing for a baby. My wife and I did almost all our research online. We asked our friends and family, but by the time we had our first, they had been out of the baby game for half a dozen years or more, and things change rapidly. I enjoy research anyway. I based this book on my hard-won experiences, and I'm giving you **"The playbook"** I built from my successes and failures, but things change, and you will need to do some legwork. Go online, find several top lists of whatever it is you're looking for for the current year, and read up on the item in question. Hopefully, you have life lessons to build from, or someone you know does, and they can help you to make decisions. Then develop your registries based on informed decisions. Because we used one of the largest online retailers in the world, my wife and I received gifts and care packages from family and friends around the world. Our house filled rapidly with many excellent tools and items to help our baby grow and develop. Many of which made our life so much easier in what was both a joyous and extremely trying time. **In the following chapter, "The Playbook," is a checklist of items** to research so that you may include them in your registry. Many of these I borrowed from Nina Spears (2022) and enhanced with my own experiences or explanations.

4

The Playbook

Recovery (Immediately following childbirth)

1. Belly Compression Belt: As her belly grows, she will need some back support.
2. Postpartum underwear / Disposable underwear: These underwear are absorbent and accommodate a larger pad. Your wife's 'situation' will likely need some recovery time, and you want to do everything you can to make that easier on her.
3. Bathrobe: Something comfortable, stretchy, soft, and functional. It should breathe well because you can expect your wife to spend recovery time in pajamas and a bathrobe. She earned it!
4. Body Lotion: Lotion with vitamin E can help soothe stretch marks and skin irritations.
5. Peri Bottle: Urine stings, so warm water can help dilute it and lessen the pain.
6. Bottom Balm/Spray: Witch Hazel Products can help the healing process and soothe the inflamed area.

7. Organic Herbal Sitz Bath: You don't want to go out looking for all this stuff while your wife is at home suffering. I went to 3 different stores in the wee hours of the morning, trying to find one.

8. Postpartum Therapy Packs: These can be cooled and placed in that postpartum underwear I mentioned, to help cool your wife's 'situation.' She will thank you.

Nursery

1. Crib
2. Crib Mattress & Protector Pad: (2) Think breathable, and I like to have two of anything that may become soiled so that if one is dirty, I have a replacement while the soiled item is washing.
3. Fitted Crib Sheets (2-4): Anything near the baby needs to be breathable!
4. Changing Table
5. Dresser: I packed away some of the clothes in my dresser and saved the expense.
6. Changing Pad & Changing Pad Covers (2)
7. Rocker / Recliner / Glider: Something to be comfortable while rocking baby to sleep. You may find yourself sleeping in this on challenging nights, so plan accordingly!
8. Bassinet / Side-Car Bassinet: Highly Recommended! It attaches to your bed. My wife picked up our baby, breastfed her, and put her back with minimal loss of sleep. This item was a lifesaver.
9. Swaddlers / Swaddling Blanket (5)
10. Sleep Sacks (3-4)
11. Nightlight
12. Sound Machine: You want something that can run continuously

and simulates mom's heartbeat. We had one that shut off after 30 minutes, and our baby woke up after 30 minutes every time. She also was a very light sleeper, so this was a lifesaver. Ours had a built-in nightlight, so we didn't need to spend money on an additional light.

13. Diaper Pail: We had one of these in 3 different locations around the house. If you keep up with them, the smell is manageable.

Feeding

1. Bottles (6-8): Find slow-flow nipples
2. Bottle Storage and drying racks (1-2): We had drying racks by every sink.
3. Bottle Brush (2) - We bought 2 of a lot of these because we frequently visited friends or family and set up a mobile feeding/-cleaning station. Also, I demolished the first couple of bottle brushes within a month or so with rigorous use.
4. Pacifiers (2-4): Try different shapes. Our baby definitely had a preference.
5. Formula: Pick one brand and put it on the list, or expect to get a formula you don't want.
6. Bottle Warmer: We bought 2 for the house and one for on the go.
7. Breast Pump: Our insurance gave us one traditional stationary pump for the table top and we bought another **wearable/portable pump** for on the go, allowing my wife to be up and moving while pumping. She termed it **life-changing**. I highly recommend it. It makes traveling easier, and she can pump discretely anywhere. She didn't have to wait uncomfortably until we got home or somewhere private to pump. She simply popped it in her bra and continued on with life.

8. Breast Pump Storage Bottles (4-6)

9. Breast Pump Storage Bags (3 sets.): My Wife produced on average 1 ounce an hour. We were constantly dealing with milk storage issues. We bought these things by the box and filled the inside freezer and deep freeze with breast milk. Breast milk is your baby's main source of nourishment, so consider it liquid gold, and keep it safe for your baby.

10. Burp Cloths (5-10): We used these for everything, and always needed a fresh one.

11. Bibs (6): When they are young, soft and made of cloth is good enough. Don't try to get hard plastic ones with a trough as that isn't needed until they are older, and our baby did not want anything hard around her neck. We were gifted a very soft rubbery one that was perfect once our daughter started with purees.

12. High Chairs: We had a stationary one at home and a portable one for on the go.

13. Food Processor: Make your own baby food at home! A cheaper, potentially healthier option than available prepackaged products.

14. Baby Plate & Spoon Set (3-4): We had the most success with soft-silicon-based things early on. Then bamboo utensils worked pretty well. Finally, soft plates that stick to the table attached to the high chair are what we found extremely useful when the time came for our baby to feed herself.

Diaper Central

1. Diapers: Get many, but in different sizes. Remember that you don't want to get too many of the same size at a time, because babies outgrow them quickly. Additionally, you can generally trade in packages of unopened diapers for the correct size. So do not open

them unless necessary. I highly recommend those with a strip that turns blue to indicate a change is required.

2. Diaper Rash Cream: Not all products are created equal, and we used one for weeks without success before switching brands and finding the new brand cleared the rash within days. Try a few different kinds, and remember to consult your physician. Apply the cream or ointment liberally!

3. Diaper Caddy (3): By the time all was said and done, we had purchased five caddies. They aren't expensive, and it's nice to tuck a diaper changing station away and change a diaper anywhere with the tools you need at your disposal.

4. Diaper Pail Bag Refills: Speaking of disposal, you'll go through many of these, so put five boxes on your registry.

5. Baby Wipes: I know no upper limit to how many of these you should put on your list. We always made a point of getting the fragrance-free sensitive wipes, and I bought these in boxes of 672 to 936 wipes at a time.

Gear

1. Infant Car Seat: We found one that was a combination stroller and car seat built into one unit, which then attached to a base. It was expensive but made anything resembling on-the-go a breeze and prevented much back strain.

2. Infant Car Seat Base (1 per car): If you find that your baby frequently travels in a relative's car, consider getting one for their vehicle if finances permit; as a matter of convenience.

3. Convertible Toddler Car Seat: Our doctor recommended our daughter sit rear-facing for as long as possible. The toddler car seat we purchased is designed to face backward and can switch,

and face forward when needed. It is designed to last her until she's 100 pounds. Do your research, and listen to your doctor's advice.

4. Stroller/Jogging Stroller: The bigger tires have a smoother ride. Find one that can hold the diaper bag too. Test it out in the store if you can. Also, measure the stroller in its closed position to ensure it will fit in your car. You don't want to buy one that is too big to fit in your trunk. It's cheaper to buy a smaller stroller than a bigger car.

5. Baby Swing/ Bouncer / Lounger: Some people do not like a "Baby Holding Area" but when they are not mobile yet, these are safe places for your baby to stay. Ours came with a lot of extra features, playing various music and white noise. It had different vibration settings and swung automatically. The seat had 3 adjustment levels of incline, and our baby took many naps there.

6. Travel Crib / Pack N Play (2-3): We had two excellent pack n plays that were breathable and safe, and they were a safe place to leave the baby for a few minutes while we cooked. They were also someplace she could safely sleep when we were on the move or away from home. We had one of these on each level of our home.

7. Backseat Baby Mirror (1 per car): We had an electronic version of this. Think of it as an on-the-go baby monitor. It was a giraffe with a camera built into it that cast to a screen. It allowed us to keep an eye on our baby when she was facing backward in the car seat.

8. Baby Carrier: We found these invaluable and enjoyed the one we had. It had a configuration where the shoulder straps could be removed, providing a seat to help support the baby's weight.

9. Diaper Bag and Travel Changing Pad: We had two because as our baby grew, we found we needed a lot more baby-related items. The backpack style was very convenient for keeping hands-free to care for our baby.

High Tech

1. Urine Sensor: To be brand agnostic, I'll just share that we found sensors that attach to special diapers that will ping your phone when there is a need for a diaper change. We found this to be very helpful. Letting your baby sit in a wet diaper for too long can cause problems. Be proactive, and prevent as many future problems as you can.
2. Cameras with motion monitors: We found one as part of the above system. It would tell us if our baby was awake or asleep based on movement. It also provided a closed-circuit audio/video feed. We loved it.

Bath

1. Newborn Bath Set: Find one with a flexible silicone bathing cup, sponge, and over-the-finger toothbrush.
2. Baby Shampoo & Body Wash: Some come as a 2 in 1.
3. Baby Lotion: We perform lotion baths at least twice a day.
4. Infant Bath Seat or tub: **"Slippery When Wet"** also applies to babies.
5. Wash Cloths (5-10): Find the smallest and thinnest, so you can also use it to sweep the inside of your baby's mouth to help keep it clean. We would douse one in warm bath water and lay it over baby's abdomen to keep her warm, and then refresh it with warm water with the flexible silicone bathing cup to keep it from becoming cold.
6. Hooded towel (3): These were extremely helpful, and keeping the baby warm is highly important. I recommend you purchase them in varying sizes. We pop our towels in the dryer 10 or so minutes

before bath time. This ensures it is nice and warm for use. Keep the hood up to prevent rapid heat loss, as babies must be kept warm throughout the process.

7. Hair Brush: Get something with super soft bristles.

8. Baby Nail Clippers and Nail File: We found an **electric buffer** that made keeping fingernails trimmed up without damaging our daughter's skin very easy. It had a light on it, greatly enhancing visibility during the process.

Health And Safety

1. Sensitive Laundry Detergent: This should be something hypo-allergenic and free of dyes.

2. First Aid Kit: A basic kit with bandages, antibiotic ointment, and pain reliever is a good start.

3. Baby Thermometer: Infrared worked best for us. The cold metal shoved under the armpit, and other more invasive methods did not work very well for us.

4. Outlet Caps: As many as needed for all of your outlets. We kept finding more outlets that need caps. If finances permit, get the outlet covers that retract without removal. A common occurrence in our house is the cap not being returned to the plug after, let's say vacuuming is completed, for example.

5. Baby Gates: We currently have 6 of these in our home. Blocking off access to stairs at the top and bottom is top priority in a home with stairways.

6. Door Handle covers: We have a door at the top of the steps leading to our basement, so that is something we had to secure. There are many shapes and models on the market. Depending on the type of door handle you have in your home, you'll need to measure to get

the correct model.

7. Cabinet Locks: You should lock up anything you wouldn't want your baby or toddler to access. Best to secure all cabinets, possibly allowing for one cabinet you designate as kid-friendly, for items with which your baby can safely interact. This encourages their curiosity and satisfies their need to explore in a healthy way. Our daughter had a very large cabinet filled with plastic food containers and lids at her Grammy's that she could scatter across the kitchen floor to her heart's content. She delighted in it.

8. Drawer Locks: There are some locks that you can install on the inside of the Drawer. In a pinch, We used a yardstick through a stack of 4 drawers to limit access.

9. Nasal Aspirator/ saline spray: Our baby still hates getting her nose cleaned, but these were so helpful and kept her breathing easily.

Nursing

1. Nursing/ Maternity Shirt/ Cover: This makes nursing in public more discreet. At home, my wife would either lift up her t-shirt or pull down her tank top.

2. Nipple Cream: Soothing cream will help lubricate the area and prevent injury.

3. Nursing Pads: Leaking happens, so to avoid needing unplanned outfit changes, be sure to have plenty of clean nursing pads to swap out throughout the day.

4. Milkscreen - Mom's been living clean for baby, and if she's built up a milk supply, she may be thinking about having a drink. Milkscreen detects alcohol in breastmilk, allowing her to pump and dump milk until it's out of her system to ensure that her baby doesn't imbibe any harmful substances.

5. Nursing Bras / Camisoles (3-4): The ones with the hooks at the shoulder for easy access.
6. Hands-Free Pumping Bra: I can't stress how beneficial the hands-free pumping system was and how much my wife appreciated it. In a pinch, she just cut a couple of holes into a sports bra.
7. Nursing Pillow: To support Baby.
8. Silicone breast pump/Milk Catcher: When your baby is drinking from one side, it will trigger the other side to leak as well, so be sure to catch it. Let nothing go to waste!

5

The Detective

Y ou'll wear many hats as a father, one of which is **"The Detective."** Often a problem will exist, and you will have to identify and resolve it without much information upon which to draw. As a result, you'll need to elevate your trouble-shooting game.

Your wife will be experiencing many changes and **discomforts**, so let's talk about that and how you can help. Morning sickness is something that, while experiences may vary, most mothers deal with in some form or fashion. Calling it morning sickness is a joke because that stuff happens all day. It can be all-day nausea and vomiting, and it's not fun. Your wife will be eating for two and probably drinking more water than ever to make her body a happy home for her baby. She will be doing this, all while fighting nausea. She will be frustrated, and you must provide whatever solution you find. There are many solutions to combat morning sickness.

My wife found **ginger chews** were about the only thing that helped, and they were safe for the baby. See what your doctor thinks, but I would stock up on natural nausea-reducing supplements because I feel like we went through hundreds of them. Also, smaller, more **frequent meals** to keep from overloading her stomach seemed to help. We went with high-protein meals that were carb-heavy. Search around or seek advice from your doctor about whatever is the best diet for pregnant mothers. I will not go into that as I don't have the expertise to broach the subject. However, I hear the Mediterranean diet is trendy these days. Consult your doctor!

Back to mother's comfort, I reiterate that she's doing everything she can to build her body into a home, or a temple, if you will, for your baby. However, her body is fighting against her, and you must be sensitive to that. Be patient with her, check in frequently, and ask if there's anything you can do for her. Even if she says there is not anything you can do, if you see that she's struggling, invite yourself to help. Ask your doctor what you can safely do to ease your wife's discomfort. You need to trust and do what your doctor says before you get too creative. We went through many different shapes of **pillows** to find the best combination necessary for a good night's sleep.

By the end of the first trimester, you should be Team Baby all the way. You and your wife should be working together, discussing what needs doing, making plans, dividing tasks, and setting up routines. Keep in mind that the mom is growing the baby inside her. That's task number one and where you want one hundred percent of her focus. You can cover a lot of other ground. I worked 50-60 hours a week during my wife's pregnancy and still managed to make sure she ate a good balance diet, encouraged her to drink more water, had a regular prenatal exercise routine, had a clean house to live in, and wore clean clothes. When I needed help setting up the nursery, I phoned a friend or family member to assist. My wife helped, of course, all while following her doctor's instructions. Still, I needed to handle everything I could manage so my wife could focus on caring for herself and our coming child. She helped with the planning and dealt with a lot of the research, educating herself on what she needed to know to care for our daughter, and I could not have asked for a better partner. But as a father and husband, I had to ask myself, what more could I do to take care of my family? I know that's what my father would have told me to do, that's what I did, and that's what I'm telling you to consider. I regret nothing.

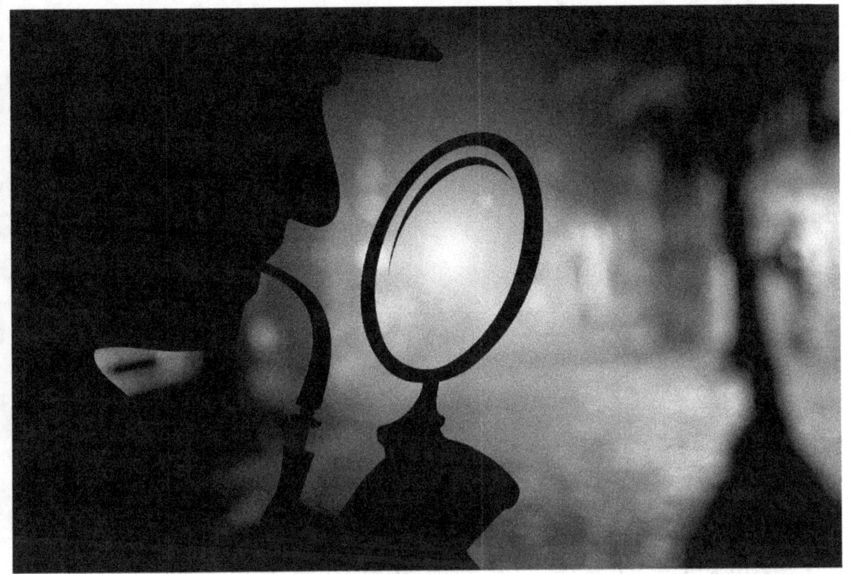

6

The Second Trimester: Weeks 13-26

By Now, you are going to the doctor's office on regular bases to see ultrasounds of your baby and check in on the mother's health. You are the documentarian, the detective, and you have the playbook, so you are off to a really great start. I packed the beginning of this book, and your journey into fatherhood this way because the more you know early on, the more **planning and preparation** you can do. You've kept your head for 12 weeks, and you're entering the second trimester now, so you can start thinking about whether or not you want to make the pregnancy announcement. I may not be a medical expert, but again, I know the painful loss of sharing the good news only to share the bad later. Let's focus on doing everything in the best way we know how. If you've kept operational security to this point and not shared your news, you can opt to do so now. Alternatively, you could wait another couple of weeks, reducing the chance of something terrible happening a bit more, or wait until weeks 18-20. At weeks 18-20, the doctor should be able to tell the baby's gender via ultrasound. Now, some people want to keep the baby's gender a surprise, and if that's your choice, then more power to you, but I am a **planner**, and I can't plan around what I don't know, so I was only too happy to learn that we would have a daughter. Also, if you were banking on a boy and thought you would be disappointed when finding out you would have a daughter, get that out of your head. Daughters are incredible, and mine makes me happy in ways I'll never be able to express. She's a joy machine distributing smiles with every dimpled squeal of laughter. So, again, if you-so-choose, you can wait until weeks 18-20 to know more about what it is you're announcing and give all the news at once. Make sure you're discussing this with your wife because she may have plans about when she wants to reveal the information, based on where she is in her career. I'm not going into that any further because I don't have any legal expertise, which you and your wife can work out between you. Just consider all possibilities.

At any phase of the pregnancy, it's crucial to emphasize **hydration**. According to (Cruz et al., 2017), pregnant women need more water than usual because their bodies are: forming amniotic fluid, producing extra blood, building new tissue, carrying additional nutrients, enhancing digestion, and trying to flush out other waste and toxins. There are a lot of different benefits to staying hydrated, such as: reducing swelling, softening skin, decreasing constipation/hemorrhoids, increasing energy, and more that you can read about if you research the issue. If you have difficulty getting your wife to drink enough water, as I did, you can add **fruits and soups** to her diet. Keep your eyes open for any signs of headaches, overheating, or dark urine, as they are symptoms that indicate dehydration. Take dehydration very seriously as it could lead to severe complications such as congenital disabilities. I'm not trying to scare you, but I am trying to motivate you. Talk to your doctor and find ways to help your wife stay hydrated. We tried a half-gallon water jug, which was too heavy for her to lift. Next, we tried using a smaller insulated cup with a handle that kept the water cold for hours and had some success. If your wife is like mine, she will only drink ice-cold water.

I mentioned earlier that at weeks 18-20, and possibly a little earlier, you may find out the gender of your baby during an ultrasound. At this point, I want to mention something about gender reveal. If you haven't seen a gender-reveal video online yet, in these videos, people do large gender-reveal events. These usually involve smoke, fire, and possibly something exploding. That seems like a bunch of things I don't want my pregnant wife around. I hate to be a spoil-sport, but if it were me, I'd tell my son to forget all that nonsense because heaven forbid something went wrong and my wife wound up injured as a result. Regardless, once the gender is known, it's time to revisit the gift registries and update them with any gender-specific items you wish to include. A word on this, though, if you're planning for more kids, it doesn't hurt to keep things a bit more gender-neutral, but that's entirely up to you. If you're having a little girl and want everything pink, go for it.

Once the announcement is made, and you can handle this pretty much any way you like, you can look at the Baby Shower. There will likely be friends or family who want to make a big deal about the baby shower, and that's okay. There isn't a thing wrong with this because a new life coming into the world is something to celebrate, and with any luck, it is a joyous and well-anticipated occasion. You may think the baby shower is about your wife, but it's not. It's all about your family, and if your wife wants to make it co-ed, then let it be that, attend, and be happy and grateful for the event. When your friends and family show up and show how much your coming blessing means to them, your attitude should be one hundred percent gratitude. Understand that although there may be a lot of 'get ready for' war stories from veteran dads, realistically, they are just welcoming you into their ranks. You're the FNG, the Freaking New Guy, and they can probably offer a lot of good advice.

Whether they will or not remains to be seen. But that's okay because you're not flying blind; you picked up this book. These veteran fathers may have a list of 'did you' questions. I advise you to take the questions seriously, and if they offer to help out with a bit of free labor, take them up on the offer. You can ask to enlist their help if they don't offer up. Pro-tip, if you ask with-in ear-shot of their wives, they'll likely get volun-told. It may violate some imaginary bro-code, but your buddy will forgive you. A case of beer or a bottle of scotch salves many wounds.

When it pertains to enlisting the help of your friends, it's time to make room for your baby. Out with the old and unimportant things making room for the new and essential. Look at your belongings; if it's stuff you can do without, you might think about parting with it. Here's the thing, it's almost impossible to overestimate how much room a baby takes. Also, realize that kids only occupy more space in the house as they age. Get used to the fact that your life is no longer your own, my friend. You're a family man, and it's time to get honest about what that means. If it's dangerous, you should consider putting it under lock and key instead of placing it on display. Find a more compact storage solution if it takes up a ton of space. So much of what we keep through our lives is just stuff and of very little importance. I'm not recommending you toss out family heirlooms by any means. If things are important to you, and you can find a way to make them work, then do so. But be realistic about it.

Before our baby even came home, we already had a sidecar bassinet in our bedroom attached to the bed. I was evicted from half my dresser to make room for burp cloths and other baby accouterments. On the top of the dresser was a bottle-making station. The armoire was more baby storage, and we had a swivel rocker in the corner for rocking our baby to sleep. There was a baby-changing station in our living room. Our guest bathroom was repurposed entirely for our daughter's baths. My wife's office/craft room was emptied and turned into a gorgeous nursery. We removed my books from the bookshelf, making room for baby books and stuffed animals. We removed some of the bookshelves entirely from the room to make space for the crib and anchored the remaining bookshelves to the wall. My well-curated library was boxed up and moved to the basement for storage. Don't cry for me; I was only too happy to make these changes because I was blessed to be a father. It's all about perspective. Don't be surprised if things that used to seem important to you, like video games or nights out with the boys, just stop mattering to you at all. I'm not saying you won't pop in the latest copy of whatever is trending these days on a whim from time to time, but keeping up will seem like too much work, and you've got more important things to do. **Congratulations, and welcome to fatherhood!**

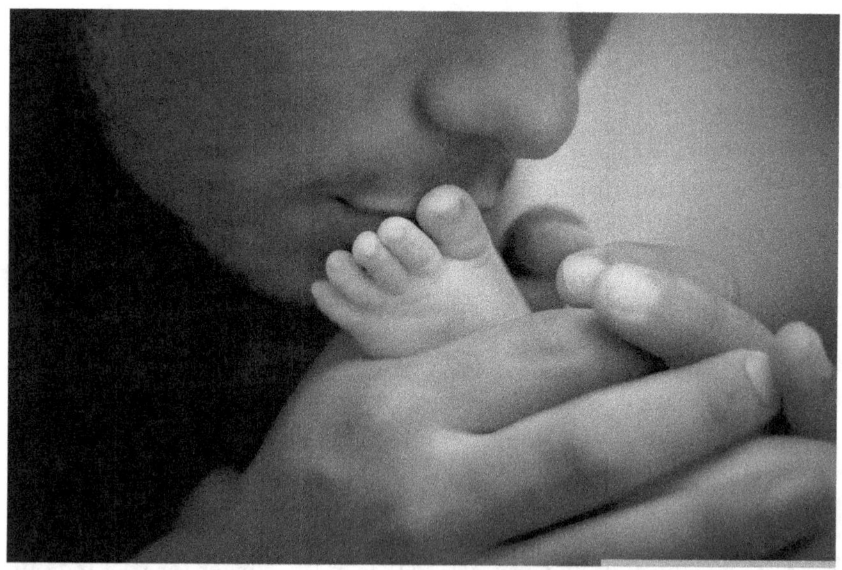

7

Nesting

Now, it's time to think about where your baby will be sleeping. My wife and I spent a lot of money preparing the nursery. It was gorgeous. We had a lot of help from my family, who have a great deal more decorating sense than we do, and pitched in, bless them. However, for a few months, until she outgrew it, our daughter slept in the sidecar bassinet next to us. You'll find that early on, you are waking up every two to three hours or more for a feeding, and if you think your wife is going to handle all that alone, you can just forget that right now, you dreamer. The nursery decorations are lovely, but if the nursery is on the other side of the house, you could make life hard on yourself. If you have any chance of having the nursery close to your room, that would be a blessing. Then, when your baby eventually transitions to her crib in the nursery, you wouldn't have to sprint across the house to peek in the doorway to check on them.

Speaking of the nursery or even your bedroom, you might consider adding some items to improve your quality of life.

1. **Mini-Fridge:** We added a small refrigerator, and I don't mean a dorm-sized refrigerator. The option we used was a 4 or 5-cubic

foot refrigerator with a separate door and freezer area. When breastfeeding, it was helpful for my wife to seal bags up and toss them inside to freeze until I moved them to the deep freeze. Having cold drinks and snacks on-hand was also a significant benefit when my wife was spending all her time with our daughter, caring for her. Place everything within an arm's reach. We made sure everything we needed was accessible.

2. **Microwave:** we added a microwave on top of the refrigerator to make it easy for my wife to have soup or heat leftovers. Mommy will have to reheat meals, because of interruptions. My wife made several bowl cozies and kept them by the microwave to prevent burns. It is very handy.

3. **Multi-purpose spaces:** The tops of dressers are great for a bottle-drying rack, bottle-making station, healthy snack bin, and anything you may need. It may look cluttered, but postpartum, the first weeks at home are all about survival. Hooah!

If you haven't already made the trip around the house installing covers in all your outlets, it is time to make the house what I call "**baby-resistant.**" No home is baby-proof, in my experience, because they will always find a way to get into some mischief you'd never have imagined, you'll find out. Bykofsky (2020) recommends the following, and I've added my suggestions from my experiences to the list:

Water heater: Check the temperature on the water heater, and set it below 120 degrees Fahrenheit to avoid scalding your baby during bath time. My water heater pushed water out at what felt like roughly the temperature of liquid magma, so I highly recommend checking this.

Lead-safe contractor: Check for and hire someone to remediate any areas in your home where lead-based paint is in use. As I understand, this is primarily a concern in older homes built around or before 1978, but if you have concerns about it, hire a lead-safe contractor.

Kitchen

1. Install Child-proof Cabinet Locks on all kitchen cabinets and stove-knob covers.
2. Store cleaning supplies high up in a closet or somewhere other than under the kitchen sink.
3. Keep cleaning supplies in their original containers to avoid confusion.
4. Non-skid pads for rugs.

Living Room

1. Apply Stick-On corner pads or foam padding that adhere to run around the edges of tables and other furniture with sharp edges. We bought this in rolls by the foot and applied it around sofa tables and similar furniture.
2. Outlet Coverings
3. Cordless Blinds - these can be strangling hazards, and if you have an adventurous child, you are likely to find them swinging on them from a nearby chair.

Nursery

1. Thick carpet or rug to cushion falls - Babies will find a way to climb out of a crib and fall over the side. Expect to be surprised.
2. Safe toy storage - We opted not to have a toy box but to use open shelves with those padded edges to display toys in tubs. The toy tubs presented some challenges regarding bedtimes, but we're

working through them.

3. Finger-Pinch guards for hinges and doors

Bathroom and Laundry Rooms

1. Kids will put anything in their mouths. So anything, if it's something that could hurt them, needs to be up high and out of reach or locked very securely away. Locking these items away may not always be convenient, but we're discussing poisoning prevention. So your laundry pods, and such, need to be securely up and out of the baby's reach.
2. Medicine Cabinet Lock
3. Toilet Lock
4. A Thermometer for bath water - I can tell you that I found this to be extremely necessary because I have very work-worn and calloused hands. According to the Mayo Clinic (2022), the water temperature for bathing your baby should be around 100 degrees F (38 C). Verify that temperature with your doctor, by the way, because things change. Keep the room warm as well, because a wet baby gets chilled easily, and keep that hooded towel close when the baby comes out of the bath; you will want to wrap her up quickly.

Whole-House Safety

1. Replace air vent covers that may have chipped or peeling paint.
2. Cover radiators and heating vents to avoid burns.
3. Doorstops may have removable caps that can be choking hazards.
4. Block access to any rooms that are off-limits with safety gates.
5. Remove any toxic houseplants or anything you don't want your baby swallowing. For example, leaves fall off plants, and it's not worth the risk of your baby swallowing one.

6. Vacuum frequently to pick up choking hazards. You would be amazed what your baby or toddler can find that you never saw on the floor.
7. Keep batteries safely stored because they may leak, which can cause burns.
8. Alcohol is poison to young people, so lock it up, or follow my earlier suggestion and get it out of the house.
9. Keep make-up and shampoos up off sinks and bathtub ledges as they can be a poison risk. But, again, babies put anything in their mouths and do not understand what is or isn't food.

Once the baby shower has happened, take stock of where you are at on the baby registries, but wait a few more weeks before you start making purchases. You'll be surprised how long after gifts will still come trickling in. My wife and I had family sending gifts from all over the country, and they were still coming three weeks or more after the baby shower. But at some point, we had to start making purchases, and when we felt we were ready, we began checking items off the registry list ourselves. You'll remember what you read earlier about babies taking up a lot of space when you get to this point. I wasn't kidding.

8

The Third Trimester: Weeks 20-40+

Are you ready? It's the third trimester, and your wife's comfort level is approaching nil. She's likely having difficulty finding a comfortable sleeping position. Potentially, whichever positions she finds comfortable are those her doctor recommended she doesn't utilize. So, again, consult the doctor, your best friend, the OBGYN. On the subject of doctors, it's time to start shopping for a pediatrician if you haven't already. You don't want to wait for the baby to be here before you start doing this. If you're very fortunate, you can search your insurance provider's website that you're happy with, located in the same facility where your wife has your baby. We were very fortunate in this regard, which meant our pediatrician could see everything and check in on the baby early on. We had a daughter, but if you expect a son, you may want to consider something called circumcision. If you are interested in that for your baby, you'll need to plan for it. That's all I will say on the subject because I don't have any experience with it. The reason to begin shopping at this point for a pediatrician is you will want to find one you like and who is taking patients. Also, getting an appointment to see the doctor may be a challenge. We had a baby during the first year or so of the COVID-

19 pandemic, unique challenges I won't share. As time went on, we eventually moved to a new city, finding a pediatrician who was also a family doctor. My wife and I see the same doctor our daughter does now, which thus far has proven to be very convenient.

Pets can be odd and may act weird, protective, or even aggressive when momma gets pregnant. Know the warning signs and how to handle them. I'm not an expert on pets, but fortunately, many out there are, so I would encourage you to reach out to them. Our pet got very protective of my wife, which eventually turned into him getting a bit bitey with her if she didn't give him enough attention. We worked our way through that and introduced the concept of a baby early on by using somewhat life-like baby dolls and the sounds of crying babies. I can't say for sure whether or not it helped because he did seem somewhat confused and a bit standoffish at first. But when our daughter came, he was well-behaved and kept a safe distance away. Our dog was never left alone with our baby; for that matter, our baby was never left alone. After all, they are animals, and no matter how much we love them, they can be unpredictable, so use good judgment. We were very fortunate that my wife could be home with our daughter. All to say that you should become informed about pets and babies and know the risks, taking whatever action is appropriate to protect your family.

In the third trimester, it's time to talk about getting the car ready for the baby. Let's get that **car seat installed**. You might as well get used to it being in the back seat, where it belongs—in the middle of the back seat, strapped in tight. Follow the instructions on your car seat, and then call the local non-emergency fire department number to make an appointment for a safety inspection on the car seat installation. I realize you probably think that it's a car seat. How hard is it to install a car seat? Don't dwell on questions like that. We're talking about your baby's safety. Most fire departments have a child passenger safety technician. They can either help you install the car seat or will do a safety check to ensure that you've installed it correctly. Check with your local non-emergency fire or police lines to see what services are available in your area.

The day you'll be heading off to the hospital to meet your new son or daughter is quickly approaching, but before the 32nd week, you need to get your **Go Bag** ready, or at least that's when I had ours packed. A **Go Bag** is just a bag, or you might as well call it a suitcase for all that you need to have packed in it; mine certainly was; that you have packed and ready with everything you'll need when your wife goes into labor. When your wife's water breaks or contractions start, you don't want to start looking around for things you should have prepared weeks ago, so complete it early.

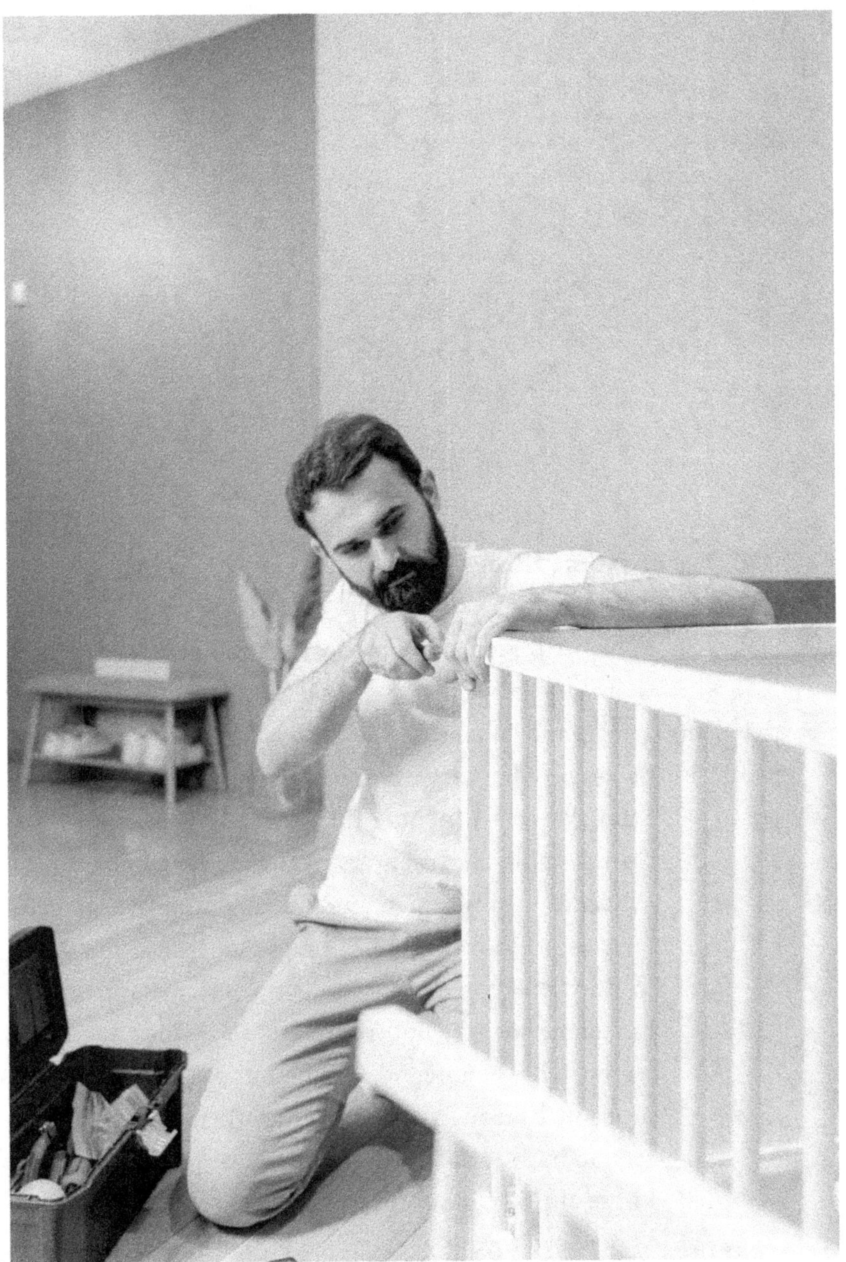

9

Go Bag

Here are some things to include in your "Go Bag"

1. Your Birth Plan - Type it up, make copies, put them in there, and be ready to distribute them. Keep in mind that plans change, and you need to be flexible so that the healthcare professionals can do what they need to care for your wife and child.

2. Stop-Watch - I include this because when your wife starts having contractions, you will want to have one available to time them, and again, you don't want to have to go looking. Talk to your doctor about what to do when you think your wife is going into labor. Remember to take notes and keep those notes with the stopwatch. A notepad will be handy as well. You'll probably be using your phone for other things, so don't rely on its stopwatch or notes app. Be prepared, son.

3. Loose-fitting clothes for your wife to wear during labor - These are throw-away pajamas that may or may not survive the process.

4. Postpartum underwear (5-6 pairs) - They make some

that are one-time use and get the job done.

5. Two packs of super-absorbent maternity pads.
6. 3-5 changes of clothes for mom, all loose fitting and comfortable; fashion is not a concern.
7. As many clothing changes for 2-3 nights in the hospital, these outfits should include Maternity Tops.
8. Nursing-Tops/Maternity Tops (2-3) - There are entire lines of women's clothing that facilitate easy breastfeeding.
9. Comfy and supportive nursing bras if your wife is planning to breastfeed. The breasts will be larger than usual. As a note, make sure you and your wife speak to a lactation specialist while at the hospital.
10. Toiletries - include a toothbrush, toothpaste, deodorant, hairbrush, hair ties, lip balm, electric razor, etc.
11. Things to help pass the time - Books, audiobooks, magazines, comic books, music, podcasts, movies on a portable device or loaded on a smartphone, etc. Remember that you need enough here to entertain two people because, for much of what could be a very long time, you and your wife will be looking for ways to relax and pass the time.
12. Bathrobe and Shower Slippers
13. Healthy Snacks and drinks (note these need to be non-perishable.)
14. Medicines that both you and your wife take.
15. Cell Phone Charger with Extra Long Cables
16. Extra Pillows & Blankets. Hospitals provide for the health and well-being of mother and baby. Father's comfort is not the primary concern. Do not plan to be anything approaching comfortable. I think I slept 2-3

hours over about 30 hours in the hospital.

17. Remember Warm Clothes in which to bring your baby home. Some like to include a cute outfit for the homecoming.

18. Baby accessories include a hat, anti-scratch mittens, baby socks, or booties.

19. Blankets and Swaddlers for baby.

20. (It's not part of the go-bag, but that car seat needs to be in the car, or they won't let you take your baby home until it is.)

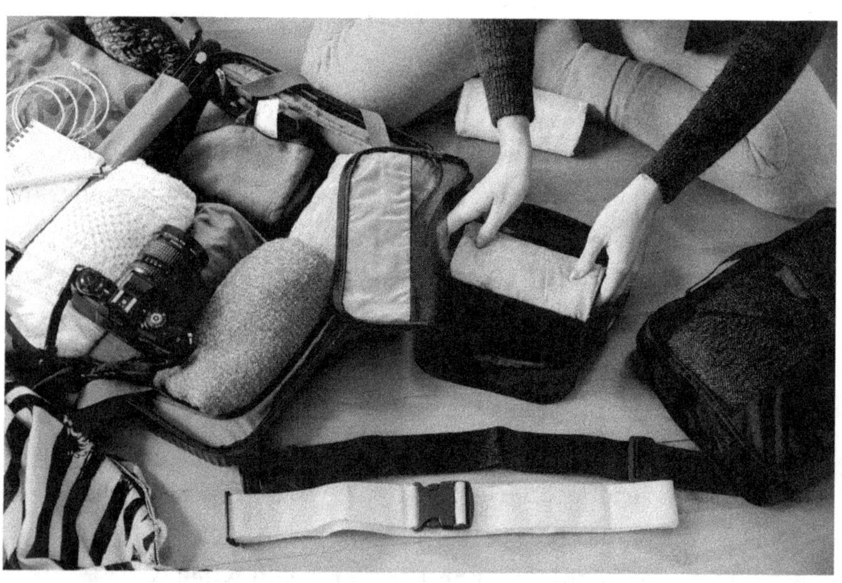

10

Childbirth: Experiences May Vary

Now, it's go-time. After much consideration, I've thought about how best to address the topic. As with the rest of this book, I'm only comfortable speaking about my own experiences as a father. I'm not a medical expert, so all I can do is share what I recall from the experience. My wife and I were one of those couples who prepared like crazy. Still, we expected that at any moment, fate would require we run out the door in a race against time to arrive at the hospital before our daughter entered the world. Such was not the case, however. My wife was 5 or 7 centimeters dilated for a week or more. Aside from Braxton Hicks contractions, my wife and I tried not to drive ourselves crazy waiting for something to happen. Braxton Hicks Contractions are intermittent contractions that come and go randomly and sometimes masquerade as real contractions. Real contractions are much more intense and come with regularity. Speak to your doctor about the differences, so you know what to expect and do. We ended up sailing past 40 weeks, and our doctor recommended scheduling a trip to the birthing center to induce labor. So, I stayed up too late, ensuring everything was 100 percent ready. I assembled all the furniture, including things we weren't going to have any need for, for

43

weeks or months. Eventually, the last of the furniture built, I loaded the Go Bag in the car. Then I triple-checked that the car seat was secured, and my wife and I went to bed for the final time as a family of two.

We woke up the following day, drove to the hospital birthing center, following our doctor's advice, and settled into our room, which we rarely left throughout the process. My wife stayed in the same bed for the entirety of the process. The process was lengthy, and I am going based on memory, and again, I'm not a medical expert. First, they administered a ripening agent called Pitocin to help speed up the labor. Much to the staff's surprise, the Pitocin worked very quickly, and my rock star wife progressed rapidly through the labor process. My role throughout most of the labor and delivery process was to do anything my wife needed. If I could fluff a pillow or make an adjustment to improve my wife's comfort, that's what I did.

More importantly, I paid attention to everything anyone said, considered any risks, asked questions, and made crucial decisions about my wife and child's care. These decisions concerned what we felt best for our family, all-the-while keeping in mind that ultimately our family was in the care of medical experts. For much of the labor process, it was just my wife and me in the room, including the portion where pushing started, and I guided my wife through breathing. At the same time, a nurse worked on a computer nearby. Eventually, I had to tell the nurse she needed to call the doctor, who was elsewhere at the time delivery began and ended up arriving just after our baby was born. I also asked the nurse to summon others because my wife was progressing quickly. I was standing in the receiving position, my hands on my wife's feet, monitoring the situation, and guiding her through breathing. I had eyes on everything as labor proceeded. Ultimately, the nurse checked the status herself and agreed. Soon after, my wife and I welcomed our beautiful daughter into this world. Experiences may vary, but our experience was pretty controlled and measured. I had done a lot of research ahead of time, asked many questions, and raised concerns when I had them. By paying attention, I realized when things were progressing faster than the staff expected. As a result, I got the help my wife and baby needed to ensure events unfolded as desired. It was wonderful. It made for a great personal story, of which I'm sharing a portion with you.

Make good use of your smartphone's camera at this point. When my daughter was born, I took a picture of the clock in the room, so I had the precise time. I'm sure you could just screenshot the clock on your phone, but wanted to know down to the very second. I took a photo of her weight and height as she was weighed and measured. A nurse was kind enough to take pictures of me cutting the umbilical cord. Everything about childbirth is a messy, beautiful, miraculous process. You're missing out on something unique if you shy away from it. I took many pictures of my wife and daughter, but remember to keep her modesty in mind at all times, as she will be in a vulnerable state. Be conscious of that. I used my hand to censor things I didn't want showing up in the pictures so that I could capture the things that I did.

We spent just one night in the hospital with our baby, who was born healthy. She received all the needed medical attention, as did my wife, and went home the following day with us. We stopped by my mother's house and introduced Grammy to her newest granddaughter. It was beautiful. Then we took our daughter home and continued to care for her as required.

Back at Home!

On day one, back home, we were thrilled to have our bundle of joy and be comfy together as a family. Although, in truth, I was a bit more comfortable than my wife, who battled many postpartum issues. At this point, those items we had on the register started to come in handy. The postpartum underwear, combined with the bottom balm, postpartum therapy packs, and Sitz Baths, come in handy. Your wife will thank you for having those handy and the postpartum therapy packs in the freezer ready to go. Healing from a vaginal birth takes time and isn't a comfortable experience. The first shower can be painful and scary, so take it slow. Maybe even get a seat for the shower to prevent any falls. My wife's legs were still a bit unsteady. Make sure you help scrub all the gel and glue off, if left on for too long, her skin can become irritated and develop a rash.

The baby is going to be sleeping a lot at first. You'll need to wake her up every two to three hours for a feeding. In this regard, you must follow your doctor's instructions, so your baby becomes used to eating. Doing this also encourages mother's milk to come in. I can't stress enough that you must follow your doctor's instructions precisely. Things change, and your doctor is in charge at this point; you are merely following orders to the letter doing everything required to keep the baby healthy. To the best of my recollection, I'm sharing our experiences; your doctor may feel your baby should be eating hourly for the first 24 hours. Do as instructed by your doctor. Remember to share the excitement of things like the first pumped milk and to make a big deal of it. Anything you can do to be the **Chief Encouragement Officer** of your household, that's the thing to do. No matter how happy this time is, be watchful for indications of postpartum depression. Fortunately, my wife did not suffer this, so I don't have any experience to share.

Ask your doctor about the warning signs of postpartum depression, and keep a watchful eye on your wife for her and your child's sake. Make sure that when your wife wakes to care for your baby, you are also awake to provide care for your wife and give her what she needs. This kind of dedication to your family and partner will not go unnoticed. Provide whatever care you can. I made formula and fed our baby formula when we needed to supplement early on while waiting for mother's milk to come in fully. When it comes to a baby, there is always something you can be doing. I washed bottles, did laundry, and made sure my wife ate and drank enough to provide nourishment to our daughter. I did whatever it took to keep her comfortable.

It is not safe to have a newborn in bed with exhausted parents. Our sidecar bassinet was invaluable here. Our daughter slept safely in her sidecar bassinet, which was affixed securely to our bed. When it was time to wake up and feed the baby, my wife would reach over and get her, grab the nursing pillow, and handle business. Revisiting the topic of not having a newborn in the bed with exhausted parents, you never know when you might roll over on top of your newborn. Go with the sidecar, an in-the-room bassinet, or any other safe solution.

Breast pumps are vital, as babies typically can't drink enough to keep mom comfortable. Many mothers will produce far more milk than the baby can take. That's not true in all cases, and I certainly don't believe that if a mother has a hard time producing milk, she is in any way lesser for it. I'm simply saying that a breast pump can be convenient to help prevent painfully engorged breasts, so you need to have one. Additionally, a portable solution is beneficial. My wife used a mobile hands-free solution so she could be up and moving around, allowing her to take care of herself or our daughter while still pumping as needed. She termed it life-changing. I highly recommend you and your wife look into such a solution.

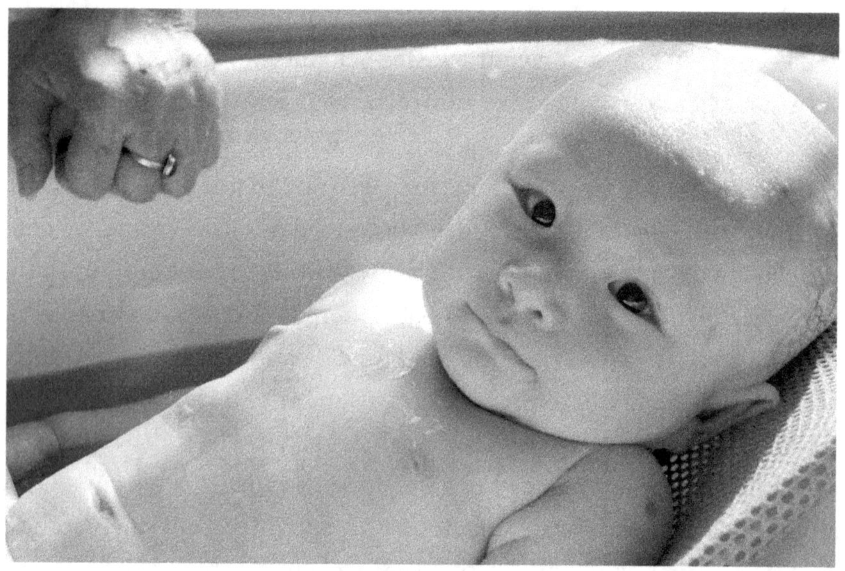

When you first have your child home, their umbilical cord may still be clamped and not have fallen off yet. If that is the case, you'll need to give **sponge or lotion baths** to keep the baby's skin clean and healthy; or at least that was what we did because the umbilical cord area had to be kept dry. Giving your baby a bath might sound scary, but in time it'll become fun. Simply lay your baby on a couple of stacked towels, and prepare a basin of warm water. Make sure you have a washcloth, towel, and baby soap within your arm's reach. Pick out baby clothes, a diaper, and lotion for after the bath. Do not be scared to really get into the folds of your baby's neck, armpit, groin, and between toes and fingers. Those places seem to collect the most, lint, milk, sweat, etc.

When the time does come for a full bath in the bathtub, safety first, and remember not to give your baby more than 1 or 2 baths a week at most, lest you dry out your baby's skin. Instead, Give your baby 2 lotion baths every day. Follow your healthcare provider's instructions on all baby-related matters. Make use of those fingernail clippers or a baby-safe file when needed.

You may expect to awaken every few hours during the first weeks and months of your baby's life because whether or not the baby awakens hungry, they must eat. Follow your doctor's advice on this. Keep an eye on your wife, and continue caring for everything around the house. Your wife requires a significant amount of time to recover from childbirth's severe trauma. It's beautiful, and it's worth it. Still, it's a traumatic experience and will take her body time to recover fully. Be patient, supportive, and helpful like you've never been helpful before. Remember that you're not babysitting so that your wife can take a nap; you're caring for your child and forming bonds with them while your wife spends some time recovering. It's the absolute least you can do. I can't tell you not to be scared. Early on, every time I picked my daughter up, I was convinced she would fall apart in my hands.

Eventually, you realize that provided you give her the support she needs, where she needs it, and hold her close; you'll be fine. It's essential to mention and always ask your doctor, but remember that when you're holding a newborn, they have no neck muscles to support their head. You've got to support it and keep your fingertips away from their still-soft skull. Utilize a soft touch and as much surface area contact between your palm and their head as possible. Hold her as close as you can. You'll get it. The doctors and nurses at the birthing center/hospital will make sure. Take every single opportunity to ask for help and information. You've got this.

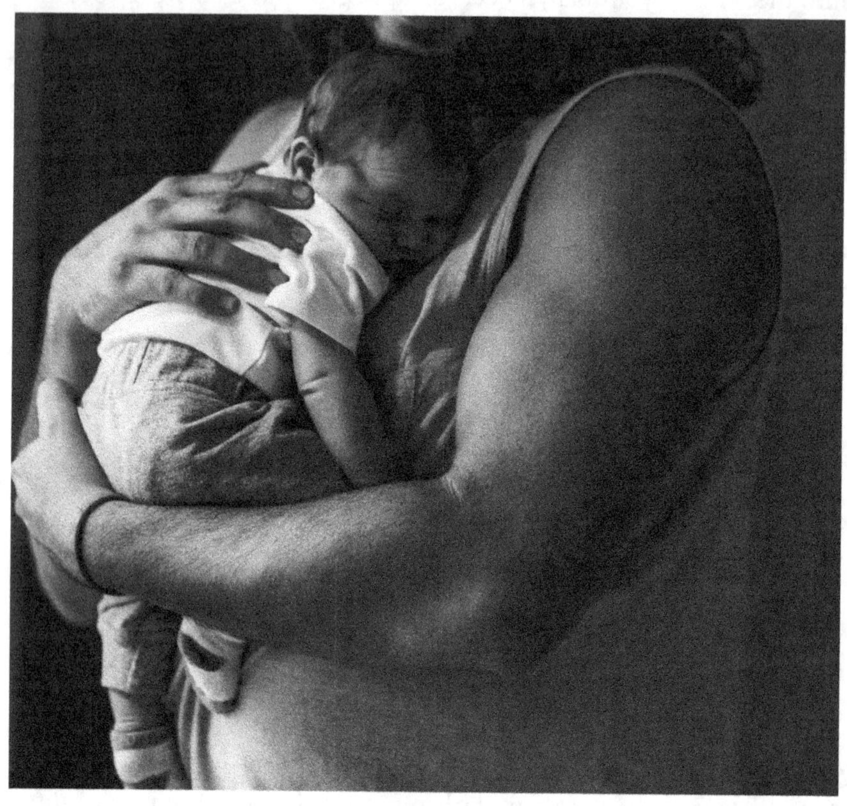

12

On the Move

Our daughter started crawling at age seven months and was already pulling herself up to a standing position by ten. On the same day she stood, she cruised down the couch. That sounds great, but once a baby starts moving, you better have things locked down. That's when the gates go up, if they haven't already. Cruising is when a baby holds onto something, such as a couch, and then uses that for balance while they walk its length. Our daughter was only content to cruise for about three weeks before taking her first steps without holding onto anything between my wife and me. We sat more-or-less feet to feet and let her walk from one of us to the other.

Some things to note about when a baby starts pulling themselves up on furniture that we didn't have a lot of time to think about, as she cruised on the same day she stood. Once a baby can raise themselves to a standing position, it's time to lower the mattress in the crib. Doing this prevents the baby from pulling themselves upright and falling over the rail intended to keep them inside. Don't hesitate on this, lest you run the risk that your child may take a tumble. It wasn't long until our daughter realized she could raise her leg, put her heel on the couch, and use that as leverage to climb up into the seat. Interestingly, she used this same tactic to climb out of the crib. Then we had to find another solution for sleeping.

The solution we found was a set of 30-inch high bed rails that ran around our bed and were set so they could be raised or lowered from inside or out by adult hands. We effectively turned our king-sized bed into a giant play yard and sleeping area for our baby. This co-sleeping arrangement had a lot of benefits and was great as far as caring for our daughter. Though my wife, who is not a heavy sleeper, did not enjoy the arrangement nearly as much as I did. It also had a noticeable impact on several other things. However, our baby was safe. Eventually, she was of age, and our situation was such that she could move upstairs to her room, where we took the rail off her crib and converted it into a daybed. She has been sleeping in her room ever since. She does not yet place the same value on sleep that her mother or I, but we're working on it.

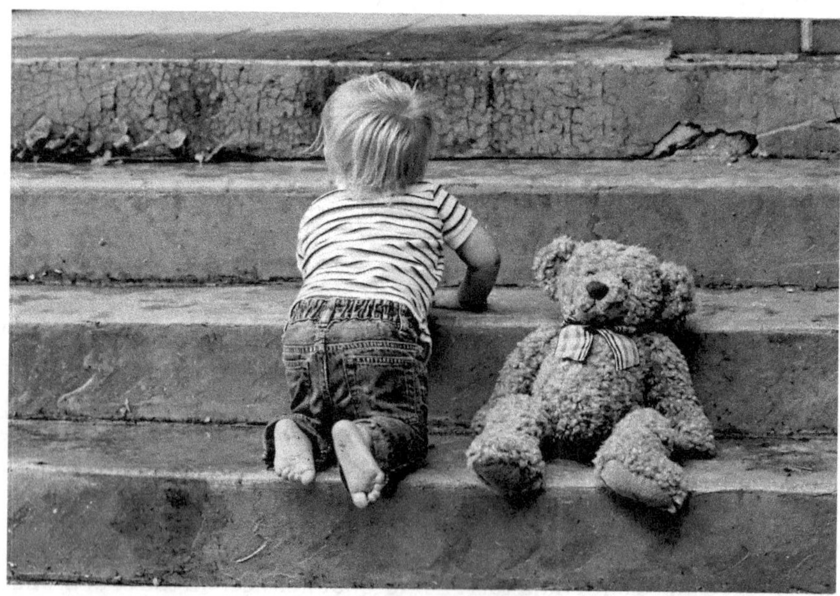

13

Lessons Learned

I know the reading got a bit light in the latter chapters, but honestly, I found that the scariest stuff was in the beginning. Once the baby is home and you start to develop routines, even though you're sleep-deprived, overworked, stressed, and always on the go, things eventually settle down somewhat. Decisions become easier to make.

For example, my wife and I decided we didn't need a formal dining room. So we removed the table and chairs from this and turned it into a play area for our daughter. The dining room gives her a view of me while I cook, and she can play and watch TV in the living room or spend time with her mother. I relish every opportunity to see her, no matter what I do. She's so very much fun to be around.

You should smile more. I don't care how hard life is; every time I look at my daughter, every time she sees me, I'm happy. I've got a smile for her because she makes me happy. My daughter is, like all children, a blessing from the Lord, and I am thankful. Whatever frustration you're feeling is not her fault, so don't let her see your struggles. Just smile, and hold her close.

You're not perfect, but neither is anyone else. Always try to do your best, kiddo. As long as you always think about what you're doing and honestly believe it's the best thing for your family and not just yourself, you'll probably be okay. Don't do anything stupid that will take you away from your family. They need you. Most problems are temporary, so find help with whatever it is.

Your wife is the most crucial person in the world to you. Your kids are a close second. So you must stay united and always take care of each other. If you disagree, do it in private, and if privacy doesn't present itself, then bite your tongue and discuss it later. Your kids need to see you and your relationship as solid because you're setting the example. So keep your cool, and always assume positive intent.

Always remember that you will set the example for your son or daughter of what they believe an adult, a man, a parent, or a father is, and how they should behave. You are the mold they will try to fit themselves into or look for in a husband. That's a lot of pressure, but you must keep that in mind and put your best foot forward every day. Never say anything you can't take back, and never do anything you might regret. Hold your family close, and always put them first.

A note on self-sacrifice because it's a fine thing, in moderation. You need to put your family first, but you also need to take care of yourself. You need to be healthy and a good, functional human being so that you can also take care of your family. So don't ignore medical issues or skip doctor's appointments. One hundred percent yourself so that you can take care of your family one hundred percent.

14

In Closing

I hope that you have enjoyed my book. I don't claim to be a medical expert, but I am a father, a husband, and a son. Every day I try to live up to the fine example my father set for me. I have tried to relate some of the lessons my father taught me to the readers of this book. This book contains lessons learned from interactions with my father and those earned in my own experiences as a father. My dad worked himself sick to provide for us. I've struggled with being a workaholic myself, and if I have a call to action for you, dear reader, it is this. Work hard for your family. Work hard at home for your family, to take care of them by building value in their lives and being present for them. Be a good employee as part of your profession because that pays the bills. But remember this, your company will replace you in a heartbeat, no matter how indispensable you think you are. You are worth more than the money you make. There are no pockets on a coffin. The real value in life is the relationships we make with the people we encounter while we are on this planet. That translates to the legacy we leave behind. Be a good man, a good husband, and a good father. Smile every day. Love, care, and provide for your family. Be ever faithful.

Thank you for reading my book. God bless your family. If you enjoyed it or found it helpful, please leave a review.

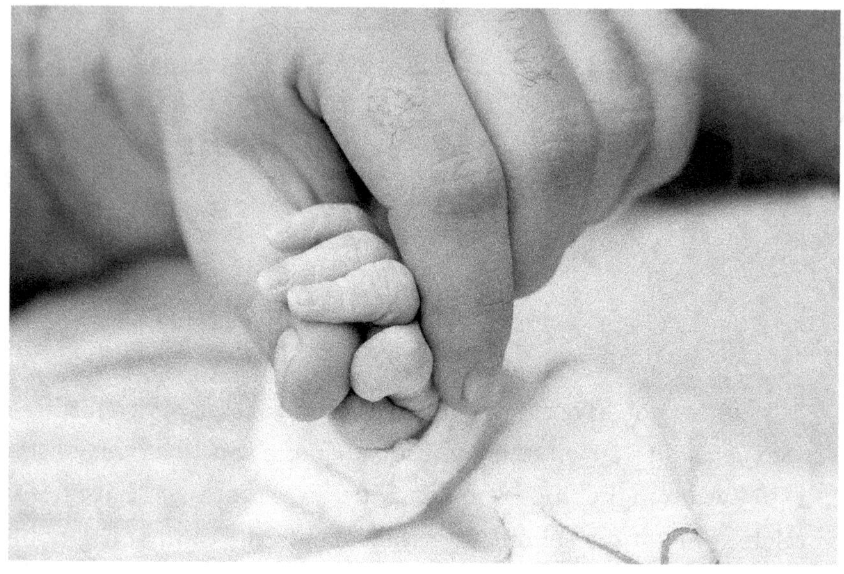

Resources

Miles, K. (2021, August 18). *Miscarriage: Signs, symptoms, and causes of early pregnancy loss.* Baby Center. Retrieved April 8, 2022, from https://www.babycenter.com/pregnancy/health-and-safety/miscarria ge-signs-causes-and-treatment_252

Miles, K. (2021b, December 13). *Pregnancy symptoms you should never ignore.* Baby Center. Retrieved August 4, 2022, from https://www.baby center.com/pregnancy/your-body/pregnancy-symptoms-you-should- never-ignore_1622

Spears, N. (2022, August 1). *The ULTIMATE Baby Registry Checklist.* Baby Chick. Retrieved August 6, 2022, from https://www.baby-chick.c om/the-ultimate-baby-registry-checklist/

Cruz, L., Cruz, L., Cruz, L., Cruz, L., Cruz, L., Cruz, L., Cruz, L., Cruz, L., & Cruz, L. (2017, October 27). *How Hydration During Pregnancy Can Benefit You and Your Baby.* Intermountainhealthcare.Org. Retrieved August 6, 2022, from https://intermountainhealthcare.org/blogs/topic s/live-well/2017/07/how-hydration-during-pregnancy-can-benefit-y ou-and-your-baby/

Bykofsky, M. (2020, September 25). *Babyproofing Your House: A Checklist for Every Room.* Parents. Retrieved August 6, 2022, from https://www. parents.com/baby/safety/babyproofing/babyproofing-your-home-fro m-top-to-bottom/

Mayo Clinic. (2022, February 10). *Baby bath basics: A parent's guide.* Retrieved August 6, 2022, from https://www.mayoclinic.org/healthy-lifestyle/infant-and-toddler-health/in-depth/healthy-baby/art-20044438#:%7E:text=Always%20check%20the%20water%20temperature,baby%20can%20be%20easily%20chilled.